THE COMPREHENSIVE GUIDE FOR GETTING INTO MEDICAL SCHOOL

From Pre-Med to Med School. Everything you must know in order to become a competitive, successful applicant. Written by medical students who were accepted to over 10 programs.

Chase A. Sawyer
Madeline K. Gerdes

Copyright © 2021 Chase Sawyer and Madeline Gerdes.

All rights reserved.

No part of this publication may be reproduced, stored in a retrieval system or transmitted in any form or by any means, electronic, mechanical, photocopying, recording, scanning, or otherwise, except as permitted under the 1976 United States Copyright Act, without the prior written permission of Chase Sawyer and Madeline Gerdes.

Cover photo acknowledgment: Banks, Clay. "Glove up!" 21 March 2020

ISBN: 9798701820881

Limit of Liability: Please note that much of this publication is based on personal experience and anecdotal evidence. Although the authors have made every reasonable attempt to achieve complete accuracy of the content in this book, they make no representations or warranties with respect to the accuracy or completeness of the contents of this book and specifically disclaim any implied warranties of merchantability or fitness for a particular purpose. Your particular circumstances may not be suited to the examples illustrated in this book; in fact, they likely will not be. You should use the information in this book at your own risk. Nothing in this book is intended to replace common sense or legal, accounting, or professional advice and is meant only to inform. This publication is sold with the understanding that the authors are not rendering legal, accounting, or other professional service.

We would like to dedicate this book to those who helped us along our journey to medical school. To our family, friends, peers, and even strangers who have given us a boost to get one step closer to our goals. We hope to pass on our collective knowledge to the next generation of future physicians.

To Madeline,
If it weren't for you, this book would still have made-up words in it. Writing this was just one small chapter in our lives, but I am excited to write the entire book with you.
I will love you forever plus a day,
Chase

To Chase,
Thank you for always pushing me to shoot higher and dream bigger. I appreciate your patience with my constant procrastination and without you, this book would probably still be in the editing stage. I truly would not be where or who I am today if not for you.
Love always,
Madeline

CONTENTS

Title Page
Copyright
Dedication
Preface
Section One: 1
Personal Statement 3
Letters of Recommendation 10
Shadowing 14
Volunteering 16
How Important are Your GPA and MCAT scores? 19
Making Connections 21
What Medical Schools Look For In Applicants 22
Non-traditional Students are the New Traditional Students 25
Best Major In Undergrad 26
Research 29
Medical Mission Trips 31
What is the MCAT and How to Prepare For It 33
Best Classes to Prepare You for the MCAT and Medical School 37
Section Two: 41
Pipeline Application Programs 42
Early Decision Programs 44

What Does the Application Look Like	46
When to Apply	48
Choosing Where to Apply	50
Secondary Applications	53
School Violations	55
Cost of Applying to Medical School	57
MD vs DO	59
Types of Interviews	62
Preparing for an Interview	66
What The Interview Day Looks Like	70
Thank You Letters	73
How to choose between medical schools	75
The Game of Chance	77
Section Three:	79
Overview of section three	80
Research	81
Get A Job	82
Enjoy Your Time, But Not Too Much	83
You (most likely) Don't Have to Retake the MCAT	84
Go Back to School	85
Still want more information?	87

PREFACE

Medical school is a very attainable desire. However, obtaining an acceptance letter is more than just correctly filling out an application. It is a long journey filled with dedication, perseverance, and honestly, some luck. With the correct mindset and planning, you should easily gain acceptances to multiple programs.

We want to take the bumpy road that we took in our quest to medical school and pave it for you. Over the past year, we tried to remember everything we wanted to know as a pre-medical student, and wrote down the answers to these questions. This book is a collection of our thoughts and advice on every aspect of the years leading up to, and finally matriculating into, medical school.

Through writing this book, we reflected upon our mistakes and the mistakes we saw countless others make. We tried to remain completely open and honest throughout this book in hopes of sharing with you the lessons we've learned, in both successes and failures. We believe these lessons will assist you in your path to obtaining your medical degree.

It should be stated early, our experiences will be vastly different than yours. Though we have tried to tailor this book to account for that, you have to live your own life and make the best decisions for you. Use this book as a guide and you will have a much easier time navigating the overwhelming task of becoming a physician.

This book is written mainly with United States medical programs in mind. Though, this information can be extrapolated for a broader breadth of medical professions as well as non United States medical programs.

We do have a YouTube channel, *Maddie x Chase*, where we discuss all things pre-medicine and medical school. This is a growing platform and resource that will have the most up to date information.

Finally, we hope this book reduces some of your stress and gives you a sense of guidance. So without further ado, grab a comfy blanket and maybe a highlighter, and let's get started!

SECTION ONE:

Before You Apply

PERSONAL STATEMENT

Your personal statement, also called the personal comments essay, is single-handedly the most important way for you to express who you are as an applicant. Many programs place significant weight on this singular essay. The nice thing is, you have complete control over what you want to write about. There is only one hard rule that you must follow; the number of characters permitted. For MD candidates you are limited to (as of 2020) 5,300 characters, whereas DO candidates are only allotted 4,500, both of which include spaces.

Anything is fair game to write about. Many people write about "why" they want to become physicians, others choose to discuss the motivations that have led them into healthcare. Many describe unique challenges, or, if need be, anomalies in their academic or disciplinary record.

Given the incredible amount of importance regarding the personal statement, you need to ensure the grammar is flawless, the sentences flow smoothly, and that it tells the reader something new. Do not make your essay simply a reiteration of the rest of your application. Bring in new aspects of your experiences, show how different experiences connect, and show how you are different than the thousands of other applicants.

Writing and revising; this is the name of the game. You should have at least a dozen different drafts, improving and simplifying each one. Have anyone willing to proofread your essay give you their honest opinion of your statement, then take those opinions with a grain of salt and make some edits. Everyone wants to help you in this process, utilize them; your advisors, professors, roommates, significant others, parents, literally everyone. You want many different eyes looking at your essay. Why? Because those people have different opinions, tastes, and experiences. Who will be reading your essay after you submit your application? Deans, professors, program directors, admissions committees, staff, and students! Literally, hundreds of different people will read your essays between all the different schools you have applied to, therefore, hundreds of different opinions, tastes, and experiences!

Your personal statement should follow a general order and style. Most commonly applicants use the order of 'Intro,' followed by three to four themed paragraphs explaining your inspirations, followed by a conclusion. However, this is not a requirement. Just make sure it flows and is cohesive. You should also avoid clichés and the overuse of 'I,' 'I believe,' and 'I know.' This will help make your personal statement sound more professional and easier to read.

We are sharing our personal statements not because we feel that they are perfect, but to give you some ideas of how to format your statement and the level of creativity you can have.

> *Chase's: Rescue Task Force, bulletproof vests, active shooter situations, and chest decompression needles are what an EMT intern deals with. Studying terrorist attacks, bomb recipes, and school shootings are what an EMT intern is assigned to do. FBI and Homeland Security briefings pertaining to ISIS and current threats to hospitals are what an EMT intern participates in.*
>
> *I grew up in a family of police officers, and I expected to follow in their footsteps. The medical field was uncharted; therefore, I think it is fair to say I have not always wanted to become a doctor. The truth is, I did not have any interest in medicine until I watched the TV series Lost in high school. Dr. Jack Shephard, the protagonist spinal surgeon, sparked my interest. I would watch and re-watch scenes in which he was performing anything medically-related. Naturally, as anyone with a question nowadays, I googled, "How to become Dr. Jack Shephard?" And that was where*

my adventure toward medicine began.

When I finished the series, my new-found interest led me to enroll in an EMT course. At the time, I was 18 years old and in my senior year of high school. This class was the most challenging I have ever taken, and I was always the youngest person in the room. We had class one day a week; Saturdays from 8 a.m. to 5 p.m. While many of my friends wanted to get together on Friday nights, I was perfectly content meeting with a study group to review the effects of Epi-Pens on the alpha and beta-adrenergic receptors of the cardiovascular and respiratory systems.

Once fully enrolled in college, I took my knowledge and applied for an internship in the Dayton Fire Department Metropolitan Medical Response System. A small office, which I still believe was designed to function as a broom closet, was assigned to me to work on various projects. Under supervision, I crafted various standing orders that were implemented throughout the city, such as protocols for active shooter situations, the heroin epidemic, Ebola patient transportation, and mass causality triaging. The amount of experience I gained was invaluable, and I took every experience as an opportunity to learn something new. I loved every day of my job and gained tremendous respect for the men and women working to protect us from the unimaginable threats to our society.

The most memorable project I led was crafting a two-part continuing education seminar for mass casualty situations. Currently, departments in the Greater Miami Valley Region utilize this instruction for many full-scale exercises and departmental training. The purpose was for first responders to better understand tourniquet bleeding control as well as "Sort, Assess, Lifesaving Interventions, Treatment/Transport" (SALT) triaging. This project was where my EMT training benefited me. I included hundreds of pictures of real patient injuries and coupled them with a specific scenario, ranging from gunshot wounds, to burns, to nerve agents. The purpose was for an EMT to quickly read through the situation, look at the picture, and determine the appropriate category that victims should be assigned to ultimately determine their priority for transport. My communication skills developed; this project required me to adequately convey a specific situation into an effective message for interpretation in under 15 seconds. The number of possibilities for treatments would seem overwhelming for most, but I thrived; my curiosity for the subject drew me in.

My medical adventure did not end at the doors of the Dayton Fire Department. This past January, I attended a medical brigade to Nicaragua. For seven days my group provided simple health care, constructed sanitation stations, laid concrete flooring, and improved water infrastructure in rural, impoverished communities across the country. What I will remember most from this experience are the people, not just the patients, but the recipients of the public health projects as well. Every single individual we worked with or provided treatment to always seemed to be overwhelmingly grateful. Even with the language barrier, I could tell that I sincerely made a difference in many lives. It is incredible that one must travel nearly 2000 miles to understand that no matter where someone is, healthcare should be a fundamental right. Likewise, I saw first-hand how education and preventative health care almost always trump treatment.

My urge to become a physician has grown tremendously since my first exposure to Dr. Jack Shephard. I have gained the values of leadership, integrity, and collaboration through multiple experiences. I have had incredible opportunities, mentors, and advisors that helped shape who I am and what kind of physician I will become. I am honored to know that my time and efforts have impacted the manner in which patients receive treatment as well as the management of future disasters. I dream of using my knowledge and leadership as a physician to not only continue to help the underserved locally but also to assist in humanitarian efforts on a global scale.

◆ ◆ ◆

Madeline's: Christmas morning when I was three years old, I woke up to a letter from Santa telling me to go out to the barn. My parents and I trudged through the snow to find a small, brown pony tucked away in a stall. As the days got warmer, I would ride her around our yard wearing a pink tutu and patent red leather boots. Little did my parents know, this present from Santa would set me on a path of endless life lessons.

I began competing at age six and got my first horse at age nine. He was young and inexperienced, so was I. We improved rapidly and soon won frequently. Eventually, my goals surpassed his abilities; while my friends were getting their driver's licenses, I was getting a new horse. I began traveling two hours north to my trainer's barn multiple times per week. Soon, competitions consumed most of my weekends. I only went to high school in the mornings and took classes online to supplement. I practiced my derivatives, wrote my college admissions essay, and studied for my first set of college midterms in the barn aisle between events. There were frustrations along the way, both academically and athletically. Despite this, by the end of my youth career, I qualified for the World Championship, ranked Top Ten in the country, and won a National title.

After I finished competing, I felt a void that needed filling. During the spring semester of my freshman year, I decided to become a certified Emergency Medical Technician in hopes of better understanding my future vocation. During the class, I found out about an organization at the University of Dayton called UD EMS; a full-service, student-run emergency medical team on campus providing Basic Life Support and transport to the hospital at no charge. I eagerly applied. The following semester I learned how to drive the ambulance, write charts, and become proficient with local protocols.

My shifts typically consisted of torn ACLs, lacerations, and bicycle accidents. One Saturday on shift, dispatch called us to our third "intox" of the day. When I pulled up on the scene, the police officer had no tolerance for the patient's uncontrollable sobbing. She couldn't answer our questions, but not because she was too intoxicated. She kept sniffling about her friend and a gun and nobody listening to her, but her words were unintelligible. The crew chief and police officer dismissed her ramblings and discussed her transport options. During this time, I asked her, "What's wrong?" something no one else had asked. Reluctant at first, she finally told me that she and her friends had been mugged at gunpoint the previous night. I assured her that I believed her and she hesitantly agreed to go to the hospital. I will never forget her looking up at me asking, "Will you hold my hand?"

I began holding her hand before we loaded her into the ambulance and she did not let go until she was in her hospital bed. My equestrian skills helped me in that situation and in turn, helped my patient. Horses cannot speak our language so the rider must listen carefully to their needs. We must use different aids to get our point across as well as be adaptable when a horse does not understand or gives an unexpected response. Many patients are not familiar with medical jargon, and therefore, physicians must explain and demonstrate to the patient using everyday terms and analogies. I have learned from horses to let go of outside preoccupations while riding. If I am stressed, or my mind is elsewhere, my horse will be my mirror. A physician cannot give patients proper care if they have an outside issue distracting them. They must be able to put aside their other attentions and focus on patients as individuals.

One of my fellow UD EMS members discovered my passion for riding and suggested I join the University's equestrian team. I became one of the team's first competing members, and before I knew it, I was elected the team's Service and Fundraising Coordinator. Through this position, I became the liaison between the team and the Therapeutic Riding Institute (TRI), our long-term service partner. TRI provides equine-assisted therapy to kids and adults with a multitude of disorders. Every member of our team must be a certified "side-helper," who helps make sure the students riding are safe and secure. The first time I assisted at TRI, I was in awe. Seeing people who can barely walk or talk get on a horse and perform various tasks that would be difficult for even the average person just learning to ride was incredible. Getting to know some of the families through this program showed me just how life-changing equine-assisted therapy could be.

Being an equestrian, I have learned resiliency, flexibility, and patience. I implement the lessons I learned from riding into my daily life and can integrate it into my medical career. Horses have not only been a sport for my youth but a passion for my life. The Therapeutic Riding Institute introduced me to an environment where horses and healthcare are deeply intertwined. Through my experiences, I learned that I do not have to pick between horses and a career, I can and will pursue both indefinitely.

Now that you have read our essays, think of some significant moments in your life that could have molded you into who you are and who you want to be, especially if they pertain to healthcare. Is there something about you that you feel makes you unique? Write about it! Is there a constant in your life that has shaped you as a person? Jot that down! When the time comes for you to write your essay you will be able to look back at your notes and skip much of the brainstorming process.

Now moving one to letters of recommendation, where others have their chance to share their thoughts about you.

LETTERS OF RECOMMENDATION

Letters of recommendation may seem overwhelming with questions such as, who do I ask? How do I ask? How many do I need? What is a composition letter? Do I need a letter from a physician? And more!

First, who do you ask? For traditional students, it is common to have letters from two science faculty, one humanities faculty, a supervisor, an academic/pre-med advisor, and at least one physician.

It is best to ask professors who you have taken multiple courses with. You should identify who you think will be willing to write you a strong letter early-on and make a legitimate effort to maintain that relationship. For example, if you really enjoyed your first-year biology professor and did well in their course, keep in touch. Try to take more courses with them or see if you can become their teaching or research assistant. Regularly stop by their office to ask questions about the material, tell them how the material they taught you helped in other courses, or just simply chat with them. Professors are passionate about the material and students that they teach. When you can show them that you took the time to take that material one step further and apply it to your research, classes, life, etc., they will take note and respect you even more! When the moment comes to ask someone to spend hours of their free time crafting a letter of recommendation, they need to be able to draw upon your character, your interest in the material, and your personality, rather than just what grade you received in their course. This will translate into a powerful letter of recommendation, not just a "copy and paste" of a generic letter they have used countless times for students they hardly knew.

To illustrate this point further, I (Madeline) am not the most gifted when it comes to physics. I anticipated this going into the class, so I sat in the front, attended class regularly, and sought help during office hours and after class. My professor and I built a strong relationship over the semester and I decided to continue to Physics II with him as well. I maintained my same strategy of going to office hours and attending class consistently. He noted my struggles and my efforts. I finished the first semester with a B and the second with an A-. At the end of the year, he wrote me a glowing letter of recommendation because he knew me well and how hard I worked to achieve those grades.

A supervisor is great for writing a letter discussing your work ethic, trustworthiness, and how well you get along with others. If you can get a supervisor who is somehow connected to education or healthcare, that is fantastic! However, it is more meaningful to get a letter from someone whom you have worked with for many years and can attest to your character over time.

Your academic/pre-med advisor traditionally writes a letter of recommendation, too. It is becoming more common for university pre-med departments to construct a composition letter for each student. This is simply a letter that consists of bits and pieces of all your letters of recommendation written by the faculty at your particular school. The advisor will connect the dots and add a little bit of their own opinion as well. Typically the individual letters used to create this singular, concise composition letter are included "behind" the composition letter itself, in case the admissions committee wants to read the original letters in-full. It should be noted that not all universities participate in the practice of composition letter writing.

An important point that needs to be addressed is 'When do I ask?' For the most part, you should ask for your letters by March of the year that you apply. Many times, the people you ask are writing numerous letters of recommendation and may have a 'cap' on the number they are willing to write per year. If you know this is the case for a particular person, ask sooner rather than later. Also, some letter writers seemingly take forever and wait until the last possible moment to complete their letters. If you are higher up on the list because you asked sooner, hopefully, that will correlate to you having your letter completed in a more timely manner.

To make the letter writers' process as easy as possible, have any forms or instructions they may need printed out and given to them in hard copies. In addition, make sure to provide your CV/resume. No matter how well you think they know you, this will only benefit you by improving the quality of the final product.

One of the most important letters you will receive is from a physician. You need to be very strategic in obtaining these letters. Having a letter from a DO is required to apply to certain DO programs, but having an MD letter is not required to apply to MD programs. If you are only applying to one type of program (MD or DO) you should get a letter of recommendation from that respective physician type. It should also be mentioned that many MD colleges seem to put greater weight upon MD letter writers and the same goes for DO programs. This means that if you are applying to both types of programs, it may be advantageous to obtain two physician letters of recommendation, one from an MD and one from a DO.

During our application process, Chase and I had very similar metrics and applied to the exact same schools. Chase's physician letter was solely from a DO and mine was solely from an MD. Chase was accepted to 6 DO schools and I was waitlisted at 2. Chase did not get an MD interview until December whereas I had 2 MD acceptances by November. The point of highlighting this is to show an aspect of the application process that is not typically discussed. Many programs say they do not put more value on who the letter comes from but, from our personal experiences, we feel differently.

The specialty of the physician that writes you a letter of recommendation is not an important factor. You should find a physician in a specialty you are interested in and shadow them several times before you ask them to write you a letter. We would recommend that if you are unsure of a specific specialty that you are interested in, shadow a family care or internal medicine physician. We will discuss shadowing more in the next section.

One final note, you should never see the letters of recommendation. On your application portal, you will be given the option to view your letters, choose NO! If you choose to see your letters, that is a huge red flag for admission committees. In a sense, it makes it look like you are not confident in what they are writing about.

After your letter writer submits their recommendation you should write them a handwritten thank you note. It is also okay to purchase a small gift as a token of your appreciation. Chase did not give any gifts to his letter writers, though I did. I gave each one of my letter writers a cookie from a local bakery but nothing more than that. Some people go further and buy more personal items or gift cards, but typically don't spend more than $20 per person.

SHADOWING

One of the hardest decisions of your medical career is choosing a specialty. This is what you are going to do for the rest of your professional life, the reason you went to medical school, and 3-7 years of residency. Let's just say, it's kind of important. There are 100+ specialties, and more being created every year. How do you find the one that best fits you? Shadow! Shadow as many different specialties as you can and while shadowing, take note of the other specialties and possibly shadow them, too! A tip to keep in mind while shadowing is to observe what the residents of the various specialties are doing. They are usually the most willing to have an honest conversation with you because they were most recently in your shoes. Don't forget, you will be a resident one day too, so take note of their lifestyle.

Nearly every physician is willing to let you follow them around. They all want to share their experiences and teach the next generation. If you are having trouble or not sure how to go about finding someone to shadow, start with the ones you know; family, friend's parents, or your own doctors! If those don't work out, you can ask your pre-med department, they definitely have a list of physicians that are willing to let students shadow. Additionally, you can blindly call physicians' offices and ask if you can shadow the doctor, or hospitals to see if they have a shadowing program. There are plenty of opportunities if you just dig a little.

When it comes to shadowing, don't feel like you have to shadow one physician for hours and hours. A misconception about shadowing is that you have to spend the entire day or week with one physician. It is typically more beneficial to spend half a day with someone. If you liked it, go back for another half day! If you didn't, thank that physician and leave at lunchtime.

Additionally, don't be offended if you get passed around to nurses, residents, physician assistants, or other specialties during your shadowing time. Be grateful and take advantage! Ask lots of questions and just take it all in.

A tip to get you some brownie points with admission committees is to shadow other healthcare professionals. We will talk more on this later but a common question on applications and interviews is why physician and not a nurse practitioner or physician assistant? If you have shadowed those other professions, you will have experiences to back up your reasoning, not just thoughts and opinions.

When you find a doctor that you vibe with, shadow them as much as you would like, remember, you will eventually need those letters of recommendation. We found it beneficial to shadow our letter writers for a half-day every couple of months. This gives you time to keep in touch, give them life updates, and not take up too much of your time. They care about you and want to know about your application process, so make sure to keep them updated after you apply! But, do not limit yourself purely based upon a letter of recommendation, you want to see as many different aspects of medicine as possible! When you get to medical school, you will have less time to shadow, and the time to apply to residency arises much faster than you will anticipate.

VOLUNTEERING

What you do outside the classroom makes up a very large portion of your application. It will be the roots of your admissions essays, your personal statement, and the conversations during your interviews. Long story short, it's extremely important.

When it comes to volunteering, you can do whatever you want as long as it benefits others, shows you care about the community and helps those in need. One question I asked myself is "Do my volunteer experiences need to be medically related?" I think the best answer to this question would be, it does not have to be, but it will be more beneficial if it were. Although anything looks better than nothing, it is strongly recommended that you are volunteering in at least one medically-related activity. I (Madeline) began volunteering at a children's hospital. Sometimes I would take a game cart around to the kids and give them some activities but most of the time I was cleaning rooms. This gave me exposure to the bottom of the food chain in a hospital setting -- a valued experience.

Volunteering your time shows the admissions committee that you are committed to helping those in need. You are joining a profession that focuses on improving lives and communities, both in and out of the clinic. They need to know that you volunteer because it is who you are, not to look good for medical schools.

You should pick something you are passionate about. In addition to volunteering in a children's hospital, I volunteered at the local animal shelter because I love animals! Through the animal shelter, I cleaned cages but I also took dogs to a local elementary for kids to read to. I talked about this in all of my interviews.

Some of the best experiences I (Chase) had as a pre-med student was volunteering at a free clinic. This was a great activity that combines volunteering, shadowing, networking, and obtaining clinical experiences. This also reaffirmed my desire to become a physician and join the healthcare field. If you were to only volunteer at one place, I strongly recommend a free clinic.

The next question that follows is "When do I need to start volunteering?" As soon as possible! This will show longevity and commitment. It would also be a great place to get a letter of recommendation. You do not have to stick with the same volunteering experience forever though. If you are not enjoying your time somewhere then why are you doing it? Try a few organizations, find one that you are passionate about, and stick with it! Admissions committees want to see you excited about what you do. It will be obvious in your application, and especially your interviews, if you are not.

"How many volunteer experiences should I have?" This is a hard question to answer. You should have a couple of experiences that you were strongly involved in. Then, you will have others that you may have volunteered with a few times; that's okay to include them, too. Try to tie the smaller things together with the bigger picture. For example, I (Madeline) volunteered at a few blood drives that were orchestrated by the pre-health honor society, so I included those activities with my explanation of the honor society itself. This shows my commitment to service throughout various activities.

There are so many possibilities when it comes to volunteering. Look for experiences with value; patient interaction, skill development, and leadership opportunities. Pre-med departments typically have organizations that they work with and can likely get you involved.

Here are a few of our favorites:
- Free clinics
- Mission trips
- Nursing Homes
- Opportunities within your clubs (even if the club is not medically related)
- Food pantries

HOW IMPORTANT ARE YOUR GPA AND MCAT SCORES?

Your GPA and MCAT are two numbers that some people think define their medical school application. The truth is these numbers act more as exclusion criteria. For example, some medical schools may not look at an applicant unless they have a 500 on their MCAT, for some of the more prestigious schools this could be much higher.

Many schools value GPA greater than the MCAT because it shows a more longitudinal academic average rather than a singular exam (MCAT). Some schools value the upper-level course grades more than the introductory courses. For example, your physiology grade is more important than your introductory biology grade. Many times students come to college and struggle for the first semester or two, this is understandable! If this is you, it is important to show an upward swing in your grades.

Obviously, the higher your GPA and MCAT scores the better. More doors open with a greater GPA and MCAT. We know many people who had MCAT scores above 510 that did not receive any interviews and others who scored below a 500 and were accepted to multiple programs. This just shows that these two numbers are not the "end all be all."

Different schools put different weights on these two numbers. For example, a DO program historically has not valued the MCAT score as greatly as many MD programs traditionally do. This is advantageous for students who do not get the MCAT score they were hoping for. There is a growing number of schools that are reducing the weight of the MCAT on their selection criteria.

It should be noted that one should not sacrifice their GPA one semester to study excessively for the MCAT. On the other hand, the MCAT should be taken seriously. If you are going to be a traditional student, many people take the MCAT at the end of their junior year. This will mean that you will have to study during the second semester of that year. Take that into account when planning your schedule and course load. We will talk more about beneficial classes to take later.

Overall, your GPA carries more significance when compared to your MCAT. Though your MCAT can help balance out a poor GPA. You should remember these are only two variables out of dozens that are taken into account from an admissions standpoint. There is a growing trend for schools to take a more "holistic approach" when screening students.

We will discuss more specifics about the MCAT in a later section of the book.

MAKING CONNECTIONS

You are entering a field that values interprofessional relationships. Even though the medical field is massive, it always amazes me how everybody seems to know everybody. Your peers in undergrad could be your class in residency. A physician you shadowed may be a member of a medical school admissions committee.

Shadowing is one of the greatest opportunities for building relationships. During my time shadowing, we met and interacted with so many other professionals, many of which have offered to let us shadow them, too. These are the types of connections you want to build. You may not be fortunate enough to have a pre-existing list of connections. Take every opportunity you have to network and build a name for yourself, even as an undergraduate. You never know who you are speaking with and how they could hold your future in their hands.

For example, while shadowing during my sophomore year of undergrad, I (Madeline) was rounding with a physician and medical student from a local university. At the end of the day, she told me she was a student ambassador for the admissions committee at a medical school that I would one day apply to. She proceeded to give me her phone number and told me she would look over my application and personal statement when the time came. My point is that even though these connections may seem so random, one day these could be the difference between getting accepted into a medical school, residency program, or even your future job.

WHAT MEDICAL SCHOOLS LOOK FOR IN APPLICANTS

Medical schools want to accept people who are going to be good doctors and good community members. This involves many pillars. The most important aspect, however, is passion. DO WHAT YOU CARE ABOUT. Medical schools will ask you about these experiences during your interview. If you don't truly care about what you are doing, admissions committees will see right through you. Do NOT do activities just because you think they will look good on paper. Find your passion.

Leadership
Doctors are not just leaders in the clinic, they are leaders in their communities. You need to show that you are capable of, and even enjoy, being a leader. Being a leader does not just mean being in charge. You must be able to work with a variety of people as well as make tough decisions. If you are in a club, run for an officer position or start a committee. This shows that when you are involved in something, you dedicate yourself to it and take initiative.

Don't sit passively in the organizations you are involved in, really dig in. Medical schools do not care how many organizations you are a part of, they want to see how you were a leader and how others depended on you. Involvement in two organizations in which you became an executive member and volunteered your time looks better to admissions committees than being a member of ten organizations and not holding any responsibilities.

Becoming a chair or executive member carries much more weight than a member who just attends monthly meetings. Think about it from this perspective: Does a medical school want to accept you to simply be a student or to be an active member of the student body. Being deeply involved in undergraduate clubs correlates with your involvement in medical school activities.

When there are elections for organizations that you care about, make an honest effort to become more involved from a leadership standpoint. Run for an executive position, or maybe a chair position. Start a committee regarding something you care about. We know it may sound daunting, especially if you are an introvert. But even if you run and do not get the position, it got your foot in the door. The new executive members and faculty will remember your interest and may ask you to fill another position later on. If you become a leader of that organization it will show your willingness to be an active member wherever you are.

Community Service
We touched on this earlier but healthcare is a helping profession. Medical schools like to see that you care about something greater than yourself. Community service is crucial in not only getting into medical school but throughout a physician's career. Make the experiences you have meaningful and longitudinal, if possible. Twelve hours of volunteering at a children's hospital over a semester is much more meaningful than twelve hours of several standalone events. Do not let this discourage you from doing these individual events, especially if they are under a single organization. We just want to make sure you are making the most out of your time and organizing these experiences accordingly in your application. For example, if you sold cookies for two hours at Relay for Life, worked a 5k for 3 hours, and made t-shirt bags for an hour but the "overseeing body" of these events was your pre-health honor society, then you have six hours of community service with your pre-health honor society. You do not need to list all of these experiences separately in your application.

Research
Something that we worried about while in undergrad was whether or not we should participate in research. It felt like all

of our peers were getting summer internships doing benchwork and we were sitting by the pool wasting our summers. Research is not necessary, but it never hurts. I (Madeline) decided to do research with the psychology department. I literally saw an article in our school newsletter about a professor that did psychological concussion research. I emailed her, with no affiliation to her or the psychology program, and asked if she needed a research assistant. Bonus, I got a publication out of it! This is a topic that I was passionate about and WANTED to do. Chase researched mass casualty incidents and the opioid epidemic with our local fire department, which he worked for. Again, this is something he actually cared about. For us, it was a lot easier to explain research that we cared about versus if we had grown *Drosophila*. There is an entire section dedicated to research further in the book.

Dedication

The bottom line is do what you are passionate about and do it for as long as you can. I (Madeline) rode horses throughout my life. I joined the equestrian team on campus and obtained a leadership position in the club for 2 years. I even incorporated a little bit of medicine into the equestrian club by being the liaison between our team and a therapeutic riding group who we volunteered with. This shows continuity, passion, leadership, and that I care about something besides just getting into medical school.

NON-TRADITIONAL STUDENTS ARE THE NEW TRADITIONAL STUDENTS

The average age of the incoming class at our medical school was 24. The age range was 20-44, 18 people had master's degrees, and 2 people had Ph.Ds. According to AAMC, in 2015 59.9% of students matriculating had taken at least one gap year. It is also becoming increasingly common for people to take several gap years, have jobs in non-medical fields, and be married with children when they enter medical school. We both felt we were the youngest people in most of our interviews. I (Chase) likely was the youngest, as I was applying at 20 years old.

Medical schools' admissions committees want to see that you are committed to becoming a physician. If you do not get accepted during your first round of applications, like many do, reapplying shows your dedication and drive. If you decide that you are going to take a gap year, it is advantageous for you to get a master's degree in a science-related field, do research at a university, or even work at a doctor's office or hospital. We will talk more about gap year options later.

BEST MAJOR IN UNDERGRAD

This is a highly debated subject! Some people have super strong opinions about choosing a certain major, others may say it doesn't matter. We believe it matters, but for strange reasons. First of all, we both majored in "Pre-Medicine" at the University of Dayton. (Yes, that is our real major and it says "Pre-Medicine" on our diplomas.) We both agree that this was the best major we could have chosen, it was fantastic! Because of our major, we were allowed to participate in certain research projects, take exclusive classes, and were the first to know about medical school application workshops. Some medical school programs actually admired our obvious commitment, versus having a biology major as a "back-up."

Other majors can also offer an advantage, such as biochemistry or neuroscience. These majors often have "pre-med" tracks that universities may offer. This could mean access to exclusive courses and specific advisors.

Your advisors are one of the most important people in your pre-med career. They help guide you by offering advice on which courses or professors are best for your situation. Because our major was pre-medicine, our advisors were part of the pre-med department at our university. They helped set up mock interviews, inform us of certain pre-med conferences, and even set up one-on-one conversations with deans of admissions of nearby medical schools! This was made possible solely because of our major.

The most common comment we received from our peers and family was "What are you going to do with a pre-med degree if you don't get accepted to med school?" This is a valid question. Fortunately, the options that we would have had in that case would have been plentiful. Our major covered the requirements for Physician Assistant (PA) school, a master's in nursing, pharmacy, or pretty much any other medical field. In addition, many students who do not get accepted to medical school on their first attempt get accepted to master's (such as biology or bioinformatics) and research programs. We knew that we wanted to become physicians and our major conveyed that to admissions committees.

Now, we are not saying you should change your major or transfer to Dayton, but if you are a first-year or still undecided, strategically choosing your major can be very beneficial in the long run. If you are a sophomore or junior and it is too late to change your major, that is okay! Just make sure you are in communication with your school's pre-med department. Get on their newsletter mailing list and schedule a meeting at least once per semester with a pre-med specific advisor to make sure you are on the right track and in the loop for opportunities.

If you are passionate about a certain subject and really would enjoy majoring in it, then do it! But understand that admissions committees may see this as a lack of commitment towards the pursuit of medicine. Be sure you can convey to them that you just enjoy that specific subject and that medicine was not an afterthought. For example, we have a friend who was a chemical engineering major and decided partway through undergrad that he wanted to become a physician, like his brother. This caused a struggle for him in several interviews, having to persuade admissions committees that medicine is his true passion.

Similar to what we stated earlier, without a pre-medical major you will need to work harder to stay in the loop with pre-med current events. You must be diligent to complete your requirements for applying to medical school. Additionally, you may not be the most prepared for taking the MCAT but with the right planning and initiative, you can still be a competitive applicant.

Another commonly asked question is "Does having a minor help?" Again, to be completely open, I (Chase) have two minors; chemistry and biology. Madeline has two minors; biology and psychology. Minors help you understand a topic in greater detail. We chose these minors because 1) they required only a couple of extra classes, 2) we thought it would prepare us better for the MCAT, and 3) because we thought it would help us stand out by highlighting our favorite subjects.

In reality, I don't think my physical chemistry course (the only extra class I needed for my chemistry minor) or my ecology course (the only extra class I needed for my biology minor) helped me at all on the MCAT. I do think it differentiated my application and I thoroughly enjoyed taking them. Madeline, on the other hand, needed to take six extra classes for her psychology minor. She truly believes those extra classes helped on the MCAT (which turned out to be her highest scoring section) and in dealing with difficult patients in medical school.

If we were to start over in our academic journey, we both would go to the University of Dayton and major in Pre-Medicine. This is what we felt prepared us the best, however, our passions lay within the constraints of our major. Medical schools want to see you doing something you are passionate about and if that means majoring in Violin Studies with minors in biology and chemistry, then go for it! It will definitely set you apart. As long as you are a diligent pre-med and can convince admissions committees that you are serious about becoming a physician, you will be fine!

RESEARCH

The topic of research could fill an entire book by itself! We were asked about research in about 50% of our interviews. People seem to either love it or hate it but at the end of the day, most people still love to complain about it. So, starting off on that positive note, should you do it?

Having research experience can do nothing but help you. Some schools require it to apply. There is a growing movement in medical schools requiring students to participate in research while getting their medical degree. When you eventually apply to residency, the number of research projects you were a part of is pretty important. One thing that many people do not know is that the research you were involved in during undergrad can be used in your residency application! This means that if you are super involved in research projects before medical school, you will have a massive leg up when applying to medical school as well as residency.

So the short answer is yes, it would benefit you to be involved in research of some sort. But this is where things can get tricky. Does the research need to be in the medical field? What about the general science field? Could it be benchwork (sometimes called "wet research"), clinical, theoretical, or even humanitarian? Well, this is where you get to decide!

Working hand-in-hand with a physician conducting medical research would likely be the most respected when applying to the medical field. However, working with a professor in the humanitarian department could be much more flexible, and being a lab assistant in the biology department will likely be much more attainable. Many departments at your university are in dire need of research assistants. You could get involved with research by simply going to the department and asking which labs need help, then reaching out to the principal investigator (PI), the main person in charge of the lab. Odds are, they would love to have your help. Just know that you are signing up for a commitment for which you are being depended upon and possibly not getting paid for.

Not everyone does traditional bench-type research though. Madeline, for example, worked on a project where she transcribed patient interviews for the psychology department; I conducted my own research on the opioid epidemic in Dayton. The point is, there are ample opportunities to become involved in research; be traditional or be creative, work in a team under a PI or solo. You can choose what you want to do!

Many universities offer paid summer research programs. This typically involves applying for the position, interviewing with different PI's, and getting accepted into the program. The program will likely pay for living accommodations as well as a stipend to cover other expenses. Most of the time you will make a decent hourly wage but this is variable between different universities and programs.

Also, note that it is extremely common to ask for a letter of recommendation from someone whom you have worked under. We think it should go without saying, be very professional and maintain that relationship. Work hard and eventually, you will be able to reap the rewards of not only adding a research project to your CV, but a letter of recommendation, a connection, and if you are lucky, a publication with your name on it!

MEDICAL MISSION TRIPS

Mission trips are incredible opportunities to serve communities around the world. They do not have to be international, but oftentimes are. We went to Nicaragua over winter break during our junior year for nine days. It was organized by the pre-med department at our university (another reason to stay connected with your school's pre-med office). This trip was truly life-changing. It showed us a part of the world that we know we would never see otherwise. It was a humbling experience and the most meaningful of our undergraduate careers.

The main downside of these experiences is the cost. You will likely have to pay for airfare plus a general fee which will include your transportation, food, and lodging while you are there. For us, it was close to $5000 per person. We fundraised as a group, which helped offset the cost.

Here is what Chase wrote in his actual medical school application on this topic:

A group of 60 University of Dayton students went on a nine-day public health trip to Nicaragua. We dedicated the majority of our time to public health and prevention; including building sanitation stations, laying concrete flooring for small villages, and helping to construct a clean water supply to a village. On the three clinical days, our group set up a small clinic in an isolated community. Our brigade saw 1,477 patients for medical and dental issues. I had many different duties ranging from assisting ophthalmologists, infectologist, and pediatricians, to teaching young children proper nutrition and oral hygiene practices as well as working in a pharmacy.

Throughout this brigade, I grew in my ability to work as a team, not just with my peers but with the local community members who did not speak English. I gained a great deal of appreciation for preventative healthcare. Many of the individuals that were seeking medical attention had very preventable ailments, but unfortunately, due to poor diet or lack of knowledge of basic personal healthcare practices, these problems manifested themselves into complex illnesses. I learned that educating individuals about their healthcare is the best prevention for future chronic diseases. This trip was instrumental in helping me solidify my desire to become a physician. I find it genuinely humbling of the physicians that accompanied us on this trip to take a step away from their hectic lives and to spend over a week in another country without receiving any form of compensation all because they felt like they were making a difference in others' lives. I know for a fact that I will one day travel to countries around the world to provide whatever form of assistance is needed to those who are in the greatest need. Apart from drawing me further into medicine, I recognized just how blessed I am, not only materialistically but in my access to healthcare or even just clean drinking water and fresh food.

If you have the means and opportunity to go on a mission trip, please do! We were both asked about this experience during the majority of our interviews. These experiences will make you a more competitive applicant and overall a better human being.

WHAT IS THE MCAT AND HOW TO PREPARE FOR IT

First of all, what is the MCAT? The Medical College Admissions Test (MCAT) is a seven-hour and thirty-minute adventure consisting of four sections; Biological and Biochemical Foundations of Living Systems (Biology/Biochemistry); Chemical and Physical Foundations of Biological Systems (Chemistry & Physics); Critical Analysis and Reasoning Skills (Reading Comprehension also known as CAR), Psychological, Social, and Biological Foundations of Behavior (Psychology & Sociology). Each of the four sections is scored from 118 to 132, with the mean and median at 125. This means the total score ranges from 472 to 528, with the mean and median at about 500 (50th percentile).

It is nearly an entirely passage-based exam. This means you will almost always be given a passage to read (typically 4-6 paragraphs) followed by 4-5 questions related to the reading. The majority of the questions tie together outside knowledge with new information that is presented in the passage. It is fairly common for the writers of the MCAT to simply copy and paste sections of complex scholarly articles to form the passages. The reason for this is to make sure you do not have any previous knowledge of that particular topic as well as to show that you can decipher what is important information and what is fluff.

Aside from the passage-based problems, you will have a few stand-alone questions sprinkled throughout (note: the CAR section does not have stand-alone questions). These questions are designed to not take much time and are based purely on outside knowledge; you either know it or you don't. This is where your level of commitment from studying shows.

The CAR section is 90 minutes long and has 53 passage-based questions. The other three sections are 95 minutes long and have 44 passage-based questions plus 15 stand-alone questions. You will first take the chemistry/physics section followed by a 10-minute break. Next, you will take the CAR section followed by a 30-minute break. After that, you will take the biology section followed by a 10-minute break. Finishing with psychology and sociology. During your breaks, you are allowed to use the restroom, eat a snack, and move around.

Now onto the topic of MCAT prep companies. There are several! Some are much better than others! The best advice we have is to talk to upperclassmen at your school and see what programs they recommend. There are courses that are taught online, courses that you can attend in person, textbook-only courses, or simply self-study with whatever works best for you. We used an MCAT prep company that was new to our area. They came and spoke to our class and it sounded fantastic! They showed us all sorts of statistics about their success rate and GUARANTEED we would score above a very high percentile. Looking back, we should have recognized that the presenters were trying to sell us something and did not have our best interest in mind. Additionally, we only knew one person who took the course before us and it turned out they were a paid representative of the program.

Overall, it was a miserable experience and made us both rethink pursuing medicine. The program was ridged and forced us into studying topics that we felt we had mastered while taking time away from studying our weaknesses. They expected that we study 40+ hours a week during the school year starting in January and 50+ hours during the summer leading up to our test date on June 2. This program drained us. After "trusting the program," studying for hundreds of hours, and taking the 14 practice tests we were required to take, both of us scored a 504 on our actual MCAT.

It goes to show that just because you put your faith and money into a program, you are not guaranteed a fantastic score. We did exactly what the program asked of us, and that was the problem. Only you know where your weaknesses lie and at the end of the day, it's your score. If we could go back and restudy for the MCAT, we would self-study. We know this is a daunting idea, which is why we overlooked these programs when we did our search. But it is the most flexible and allows you to use a variety of resources from any company you want! There are plenty of "skeleton schedules" online that you can pull from and customize for you as well as tons of free practice questions from top companies!

Now when we say self-study, we do not mean opening up your old biology textbook and start reading. Buy one of the big-name MCAT prep books and work through it. If you are a biochem major, do you really need to spend the majority of your time studying biochem? We would imagine not! Study your weaknesses. Take several practice tests and review them question by question. Learn the material from MCAT practice questions, not from reading textbooks. This will allow you to actively learn and be much more time-efficient.

The next question is when do you start studying? To answer this question you should first ask yourself when are you taking the test? We would not recommend taking your test during the school year, but rather a couple of weeks after you finish classes in the spring before you apply (May or early June). This way you can start chipping away at the material starting in January and gradually ramp up your studies throughout the semester. Then, dedicate the few weeks at the beginning of summer break to study, transitioning to mainly practice problems. You should try to take several full-length practice tests (5-7). Taking timed tests similarly to test day will build mental endurance. Additionally, it is shown that the more practice questions we do, the more we learn and retain in a shorter period of time.

Strategically schedule your course work to help you in your MCAT studies. We would recommend taking biochemistry either the semester you are studying for the MCAT or the semester before. Biochemistry is the highest yield subject of the test. Additionally, we have heard about some students taking the semester off to study for the MCAT, you do not need that long of a study period. But, definitely take a lighter course load that semester to minimize stress. Study strategically and efficiently and you should do well!

The day of your exam should not feel new to you. By completing several practice tests and simulating a real testing environment it should feel like any other day of studying. In the week leading up to your actual test, go to sleep and wake up at the same time every day. Eat basic foods; you do not want to get food poisoning the day before. Eat the same food you are going to eat during your test-day breaks around the same time that your actual breaks are going to be. To put it simply, reduce the number of variables that you are going to deal with. The only variable you want to have is the test, not an illness or upset stomach.

BEST CLASSES TO PREPARE YOU FOR THE MCAT AND MEDICAL SCHOOL

As you probably now know, MCAT scores are very important in ruling out applicants who fall below a school's MCAT minimum. Put plainly, your MCAT score can close doors, regardless of who you are as a person. Hate it or love it, it's required so try your best and recognize the opportunity you have to capitalize with a great score.

If we could stress the importance of one subject for this test, it would be biochemistry. Biochem is explicitly stated in sections one and two, however, it is everywhere on the MCAT! We are not joking when we say that during the MCAT we had biochemically related passages in the CAR and psychology sections. The authors of the test love to add biochem questions wherever they can. If you focus on one subject, focus on biochemistry!

Here is a list of the classes you should definitely take before taking the MCAT:

- 2 semesters of General Biology
- 2 semesters of General Chemistry
- 2 semesters of Organic Chemistry
- 2 semesters of General Physics
- 1 semester of Biochemistry
- 1 semester of General Psychology
- 1 semester of General Sociology

Here is a list of upper-level classes that would be useful to take before the MCAT

- Molecular Cell Biology

- Microbiology
- Physiology
- Genetics

Some people may argue that you need anatomy for the MCAT but neither of us recall ever having an anatomy question, even during practice. Don't try to cram anatomy in before the MCAT, but take it before going to medical school!

Additionally, here are our schedules from undergrad:

	Chase's	Madeline's
Summer 2013	Introduction to Engineering Design	
Fall 2013	Chinese I	Chinese I
Spring 2014	Chinese II	Chinese II
Summer 2014	Principles of Engineering	
Spring 2015	Community Leadership Environmental Science	Environmental Science English I
Summer 2015	Human Biology General Psychology	
Fall 2015	General Chemistry I + Lab Intro Math for Engineering Calculus I English I Statistics	Concepts of Biology I + Lab General Chemistry I + Lab Calculus I Intro to Religion and Theory
Spring 2016	General Chemistry II + Lab Introduction to Literature Engineering Tech Project EMT Lecture + Lab	(Retake) General Chemistry I Philosophy 101 Concepts of Biology II + Lab Oral Communication Calculus II EMT Lecture + Lab
Summer 2016	Intro to Philosophy English Composition II	General Chemistry II
Fall 2016	Concepts of Biology I + Lab Organic Chemistry I + Lab History (West and the World) Calculus II	Statistics Organic Chemistry I + Lab History (West and the World) Physiology I General Chemistry II Lab

Spring 2017	Concepts of Biology II + Lab Organic Chemistry II + Lab Oral Communication History (19th Century Africa) Social Sciences	Biopsychology Organic Chemistry II + Lab Extreme Physiology History (19th Century Africa) Social Sciences Child psychology
Fall 2017	General Genetics Physiology I Mission Trip Physics I + Lab Intro to Religion and Theory Principle of Sociology	General Genetics Physiology I Mission Trip Physics I + Lab Psychology Elective Principle of Sociology
Spring 2018	General Microbiology Biochemistry Writing for Health Professions Pre-Med Capstone Physics II	General Microbiology Biochemistry Writing for Health Professions Pre-Med Capstone Physics II
Summer 2018	Take MCAT	Take MCAT
Fall 2018	Physiology Lab Human Anatomy Physical Chemistry Biochemistry Lab Piano I Medical Ethics Darkroom photograph	Physiology Lab Human Anatomy Developmental Psych Biochemistry Lab Painting Medical Ethics
Spring 2019	Abnormal Psychology Ecology Immunology Medical Terminology Islamic philosophy and Culture Microbiology Lab Physics II Lab	Abnormal Psychology Ecology Immunology Medical Terminology Islamic philosophy and Culture Microbiology Lab Physics II Lab

Technically, there are no prerequisites required for taking the

MCAT but just remember that there are requirements for being accepted into most medical schools. With this being said, some may ask "Do I need to take any of these classes to do well on the MCAT?" The short answer is no, but it would help. If you have never heard of an amino acid, how would you expect to understand it on a practice question? Though, there are some MCAT preparation companies whose textbooks and videos cover nearly all the knowledge necessary to succeed on this exam.

SECTION TWO:

The Application process

PIPELINE APPLICATION PROGRAMS

This is not the same thing as the "early decision programs." The early decision programs will be discussed in the next section. There are basically three different programs that fall under the blanket term of "pipeline application programs":

The easiest of these to understand is called by many different names. The general concept is medical schools accept students into their program during their junior year of undergrad. This type of program allows you to apply to medical school during your junior year before you even take the MCAT! They use your ACT or SAT score and your undergraduate GPA. If accepted, students are typically exempt from taking the MCAT and just need to maintain a certain GPA until they graduate. This is our favorite and one we wished we knew about before applying! Ask your pre-med department if they are aware of any programs like this. You can find more information about these programs by searching various school's websites for alternative applications to their medical school.

Another common program that many schools offer is a master's degree that guarantees an interview at their associated medical school. This is a great option if you are unsure of your desire to go to medical school, do not think you are competitive enough, or decided on medicine later on. This type of program will typically put you in many of the same classes as the medical students. This is to see how well you perform at that level. This path could also have research integrated into the program. This is very beneficial not only for your medical school application, but to eventually help you in your residency applications, too!

The final path typically happens by accident or coincidence. It is when you attend an undergrad institution that has a medical school affiliation. For example, the University of Dayton has a partnership with Marian University's school of medicine. If you are a student at UD and have above a certain GPA and MCAT, you are guaranteed an interview at Marian! This is relatively common and your school may have some form of partnership with a medical school, too. Hence, another reason to make sure you are in constant communication with your pre-med department. On a similar note, these programs do not have to be two separate schools, it could be that your undergrad university also has a medical school. Many medical schools reserve a certain number of seats for students that graduate from their "home institution." This can be as high as fifty percent!

The point of this section is to inform you of the lesser-known paths to take to get into medical school. If you play your cards right you may not have to take the MCAT or interview at multiple institutions. You could even have an advantage at your home institution's medical program! Make sure to talk to your pre-med advisor to see if they know of any programs like these!

EARLY DECISION PROGRAMS

The early decision program is very unique and there are strict guidelines that must be followed; you are only permitted to apply to ONE medical school, you must apply before August 1st, and you are required to attend that school if accepted. If you are not selected, you can apply to as many other schools as you wish but you may not hear back until as late as October 1st.

This is extremely risky, and normally only the most competitive students even think of attempting this type of application. Schools accept a small percentage of the early decision program applicants. There are benefits to this program, however. It shows your favorite school that you are very serious about wanting to matriculate into their program, especially if you have a good reason (i.e. your spouse is already in the program). In addition, your application will be one of the first they will look at during the cycle. Note that in the application process, there are typically questions allowing you to explain these special circumstances in the traditional secondary application.

We want to be clear when saying this; we do NOT recommend applying in this manner for several reasons. First, even if you are a competitive applicant your chances of acceptance are still slim. Second, if you are rejected you are left to apply late in the application cycle for other schools. We will talk more about this later, but this is one of the worst things you can do to your application. Finally, the risk versus reward is just too high. If you are already an incredible applicant, your chances of acceptance are just slightly higher at a specific school without applying via this program. Additionally, you will have a greater chance of being accepted at other schools as well because you have applied sooner rather than later to all of them. If you are truly contemplating this route, please just seriously consider all potential outcomes, both positive and negative.

WHAT DOES THE APPLICATION LOOK LIKE

The application to medical school is a very similar format to the one many of us used for applying to undergrad. It is a single, lengthy questionnaire that asks about everything from parental income to extracurricular activities.

There are two application platforms; AMCAS and AACOMAS. AMCAS is the application service for allopathic (MD) schools and AACOMAS is the application service for osteopathic (DO) schools. We explain the difference between these programs later in the book but before you apply you need to decide which program you want to apply to. Many medical students, including us, apply to both. This just means that you will fill out the AMCAS application as well as the AACOMAS application. They are very similar so many times you can just copy and paste your answers between the two.

All medical schools within either AMCAS or AACOMAS share the same primary application. Once it is completely filled out, you must input which schools you would like your application sent to. You will also send your transcripts to these platforms so all of the schools you apply to can see them here. This prevents you from having to send them individually to all of the schools. We will talk about the cost of all of this later! In addition to you submitting items to these platforms, you will also have those writing your letters of recommendation submit their letters here, too.

The application is easy to fill out for the most part but as we said earlier, it is long. It is a culmination of everything you have done prior to medical school. Even though you submit your transcripts, you must manually input your classes into the application and the grades you received. We found starting to fill it out early and working on it little by little was helpful!

WHEN TO APPLY

The primary application will open as early as April. You should start to complete the initial essays and questionnaire during this time. The actual submit button will not become available until late May or early June. You should have your application ready to submit when it opens. If you only listen to one piece of advice in this book, please SUBMIT YOUR APPLICATION AS SOON AS POSSIBLE!

If your name is at the top of the application list you are much more likely to be asked to interview than if you are in the middle or bottom. During the early stages of the application cycle, admissions departments are much more lenient in their selection criteria. Once interviews start (August), the committee will have real applicants whom they have met and interacted with stuck in their minds. If your application does not REALLY stand out, you will likely be pushed to the "maybe later" pile. Think about it, if you apply later in the cycle (anytime after July) there are fewer spots open. Therefore, they will only select the best applicants to fill the few remaining spots.

Another reason to apply early is that it shows your willingness to submit items before the deadline, showing the selections committee that you are responsible and eager without even opening your application! Why would they want a student who doddled with their application three months after it opened? Trust us, press submit on the day it opens and your chances are greatly improved.

One common question regarding submitting the application is whether or not you should wait to get your MCAT score back (which takes about 30 days from the test day). You can, and we believe you should, submit your primary application before you receive your MCAT score. We actually took our MCAT on June 2nd, and submitted our primary applications on June 3rd. Before we even took the MCAT we decided that regardless of what our scores were, we were applying no matter what. As you already know, we both received 504s, a score neither of us was comfortable with. However, as many of you also know, both of us received several interview invitations and acceptances before some of our peers even submitted their primary applications!

Many people may feel strongly about wanting to see their scores before hitting submit because if they do not score where they would like, they plan to retake the test. First of all, go into your MCAT planning to only take it once. It is a time-consuming process that should not be repeated if you can help it. Secondly, if you wait and decide to retake the MCAT, you will submit late, decreasing your chances of acceptance. Even if you get a score you are comfortable with, but decided to wait and see your actual score before submitting, you still delayed submission of your application! On a positive note, some schools will still send you their secondary application even if they have not received your MCAT scores.

To put this point into perspective, we have several friends who were fantastic applicants with great volunteering and leadership experiences, lots of research, 3.7+ GPAs, and 90+ percentile on their MCATs who applied in September. A few were waitlisted late in the year and many did not even get an interview invitation. They spent thousands of dollars on their applications all for nothing. Now if they would have applied in early June, we would almost guarantee they would have been accepted at some of their top choices. Do yourself the easy favor and apply as soon as you can.

CHOOSING WHERE TO APPLY

When we were applying we didn't realize that it was possible to apply to the *wrong* schools. Not knowing what to look for in a program significantly reduces your chance of being accepted. There are several factors that you need to consider when applying. These include in-state vs out-of-state, private vs public, MD vs DO, mission statements, and Caribbean.

In general, the average student has the greatest probability of being accepted to an in-state, public, DO program. Let us expand on this. Many programs have a mandatory quota to reach regarding the number of students from its residing state. This is especially true for public programs but many private schools will also need to satisfy a specific number of students from their particular state as well. This basically boils down to government grants. In a sense, the government says "For us to give you grants you must accept at least X% of students from your state." This is commonly around 50% but can vary greatly. For example, Florida State University likes its class to be made up of about 95% Florida residents.

We were fortunate because Ohio has *eight* medical schools. Some states aren't so rich with programs but luckily the more plentiful states tend to share the wealth in this regard. For example, applicants living in Kentucky or Indiana may get "in-state" status for some schools in Ohio; it could be any applicant from those states or maybe just those residing in a few neighboring counties. Either way, every school will be different but make sure to keep an eye out for these opportunities.

Public schools are generally easier to get accepted into. Private programs are known to be more elite. This is a generalization, but nevertheless, it holds true more times than not. Additionally, just because a school is public does not mean it is going to be less expensive; more on this later.

As we will discuss later in the book, DO programs typically have lower MCAT and GPA requirements. Thus, they are more obtainable if you have lower metrics. In this case, you may want to apply to a greater number of DO programs than MD.

One factor that we did not look into when applying (that we should have) was reading the mission statement of each school before submitting our primary applications. To portray this point, let us explain our mistake. When we were applying, we applied to nearly every school in Ohio and the nearby states. There are two schools in these states that have mission statements that clearly emphasize their goal of increasing the number of physicians who are underrepresented minorities in the United States; we are both white, non-Hispanic, and from the suburbs. When we received their secondary applications, one question asked what underrepresented minority group do we associate with and how this has impacted our lives. Only then did we look at their mission statements and realize that we had very little chance to matriculate into their program. The point of reading these short three sentence mission statements is to make sure you are actually a student they are interested in and you do not waste your money. If you are from an underrepresented minority group, then you should be on the lookout for programs like these! If you are not, then realize you will likely not be considered a priority to their admissions committee.

Caribbean schools are typically the easiest programs to get accepted into as they have massive class sizes (2-4x larger than U.S. programs) and typically lower MCAT and GPA requirements. The major downside to these programs is you will have a greatly reduced probability of getting a residency spot in the United States, especially if you want to go into something competitive (surgery, dermatology, etc.). In addition, you will not have the level of attentiveness from faculty that smaller programs have to offer. Finally, many of the schools are 'for profit,' thus the dollar typically comes before the student. We know a few people who have taken this route; one got a fantastic residency spot and the other had to take a gap year after medical school. To be blunt, we would not consider a Caribbean program, though studying on an island would be nice.

The best resource we found for comparing medical schools is AAMC's *Medical School Admission Requirements (MSAR)*. Note, this is only for allopathic programs. Other than that this resource is fantastic! You can filter schools based on MCAT scores, GPAs, location, and more! It can look at specific schools to see what their class sizes look like, what states their students typically come from, and find their mission statements, too. You will also be able to find who is considered "in-state" at each school. It does cost a little money but it was well worth it!

SECONDARY APPLICATIONS

Almost every school will have a secondary application. Some schools will send you an email within hours of submitting your initial application while others won't send it to you for months. These can be as easy as completing one 500-character essay or as complex as asking you to take another standardized test (most likely the CASPer test: a short-ish online character assessment) and completing 10 additional essays. Do not worry though, these essays are typically similar between various schools.

When you receive a secondary application, try to complete and return it as soon as possible (no longer than two days). To help cut down on time, create a master document where you keep the essays from all of your applications. You will undoubtedly be able to reuse some of your responses for multiple schools with just minor tweaks.

Here are several examples of essays you may be asked on your secondary applications:
- What are your greatest strengths and why?
- Describe your most influential volunteer experience and why?
- Describe any circumstances adversely affecting your academic performance.
- Provide the names, dates, and departments of physicians you have shadowed.
- Why do you want to be a student at our medical school?
- Describe your motivations for wanting to become a physician.
- Why do you want to be a DO compared to an MD?
- What specialty do you think you want to practice?
- Why do you want to serve in rural or underserved

areas?
- Please share anything else you would want the admissions committee to know.

Most of the time you are limited to a character count, you will likely use all of them. Sometimes the number of characters allotted is minimal and you will need to be concise. Other times, you will have unlimited space. When you are writing your responses, make sure to review that school's website for their mission and values so you can tailor your responses accordingly.

From a financial point of view, be prepared for the additional cost. Secondary applications nearly always have an additional application fee ranging from $50-$100 per school. More on finances in the next section!

SCHOOL VIOLATIONS

READ AT LEAST THE FIRST PARAGRAPH!

Regardless of whether you have violations or not, the first paragraph of this section is for you. Your social media pages WILL play a role in your application. We intentionally kept our social media pages public because neither one of us post much more than our favorite hiking views and holidays with our families. We knew that we would *benefit* from admissions committees seeing photos of us passing the football with our younger brothers. We know that not everyone is in the same boat. We are not telling you to delete your social media and start from scratch. Just please be cognizant of what you are posting. You may not have any school violations but many of you likely have photos of underage drinking on your profiles right now. At the very least make your profiles private and ensure that what is visible to the public paints you positively. We are stepping off of our soapbox now.

Moving onto school violations; these have the potential to ruin your application. They also may not be a big deal. You will need to disclose any school violations on your primary application to medical school. You can not hide this from them, thus the best way to prevent a medical school from seeing a violation is to not have one!

Violations such as underage drinking are typically overlooked for the top tier applicants who are one-time offenders. But for the less competitive applicants, it is a red flag. It shows the admissions committee that you do not respect the rules and can be reckless. Do they want a student representing their school and hospital to be a rule-breaker? Probably not.

Though, there is good news; a lot of applicants have drinking violations. Oftentimes this is a one-time offense for students in their freshman year. Although this does not make it okay in the admissions committee's eyes, it is less concerning because it is so common. Now there are major violations, such as academic dishonesty or sexual allegations, that will pretty much kill your application. I'm not even sure if a medical program would look at your application if these are on your file.

Every medical school will perform a full background check and some programs will run a credit check on you. This is to make sure you are not a sex offender or have a 400 credit score (showing your responsibility, or lack thereof). Simple issues such as traffic tickets will be okay. Though, again, if you have something major like intent to sell an illicit substance, these may jeopardize your ability to matriculate. One final note, many medical schools have the ability to drug test their students; oftentimes this occurs before students matriculate. Just be aware of that.

COST OF APPLYING TO MEDICAL SCHOOL

The cost associated with the entire application process can be pretty daunting. You will need to have a plan, especially if you are paying for this yourself as a college student like we did. Here is the breakdown of approximately how much it will cost to apply to medical school based on our 2018 experience:

MCAT study resources: $0-$10,000
MCAT fee: $320 + travel + rescheduling fees (if need be -- Chase rescheduled twice)
Primary application MD: $170 for the first school and $40 for each additional school
Primary application DO: $196 for the first school and $46 for each additional school
Secondary applications: $50-$100 per school.
Interview: Cost of travel + thank you letters

In our opinion, you should not let the cost of applying to medical school stop you. When you are applying, do not limit the number of schools you are applying to just because it is expensive. You need to cast a wide net. Most advisors recommend 10-15 schools; we initially applied to 21 and then decided to complete 17 secondary applications. This was partially because increasing the number of schools we applied to increased the probability of getting accepted into the same program. In hindsight, we do not regret applying to so many schools, it was a safety factor and helped reduce our anxiety. Though, it did hurt our bank accounts.

Now speaking of money, how much did it cost? Chase spent $1881.49 for the whole application process (not including the

MCAT prep course and exam costs). However, we were extremely frugal on travel expenses. We drove to interviews the day of if possible, stayed in the cheapest AirB&B, and took the cheapest flights.

Regarding additional fees, Chase rescheduled his MCAT twice, which cost $95 each time. Also, his MCAT studying resources cost $1,999 (which was a huge waste of money in his humble opinion). My MCAT studying resources cost $2,799 (which was definitely not the best use of my money).

One key cost that many people do not factor in is the cost of their actual bachelor's degree, but that is a worry for another day. So, overall applying to medical school is expensive. You will need to plan accordingly for the several thousands of dollars you will ultimately spend. Both of us worked for our university during undergrad. I also had a paid research position. Both of these activities look great on applications and can help offset the cost of applying.

On a related topic, we would not pay for these items with a credit card if you cannot confidently pay off the balance. You can have your acceptance letters from medical school revoked if you have poor credit. Though this is extremely rare, we would recommend trying to not even make that a possibility.

MD VS DO

There are two types of physicians in the United States, MDs and DOs. This means that they obtained either a Doctor of Medicine degree or a Doctor of Osteopathic Medicine degree, respectively. Regardless of which two letters someone has at the end of their name, they are still a physician and addressed as "Doctor."

There are many more similarities than differences between these two degrees. The main differences being the overall approach and additional training in Osteopathic Manipulative Medicine (OMM) that DO students must complete. Learning this practice adds about 200 more hours of training for these students than their MD counterparts. Osteopathic programs also teach a more holistic approach to diagnosing a patient's condition and are less inclined to rely on pharmaceuticals to treat a patient long term.

Both programs must complete two board exams during medical school, one after their second year and one after their third year. Osteopathic boards are about 30% longer than allopathic due to additional questions regarding OMM. In the past, osteopathic students have opted to take both allopathic and osteopathic board exams in order to make them more competitive during residency application. This is a hot topic right now and seems to be continuously evolving, so if you are considering applying to osteopathic programs be sure to keep up on this matter.

A major difference for applicants is the application portal for medical school. Allopathic program applications are through the American Medical College Application Service (AMCAS) and osteopathic program applications are through the American Association of Colleges of Osteopathic Medicine Application Service (AACOMAS). These applications are nearly identical; the main difference is the personal statement length and some additional work on your part. As stated in the first section, as of 2020, MD candidate's personal statements are limited to 5,300 characters whereas DO candidates are only allotted 4,500, both include spaces. Additionally, the two application portals do not communicate with each other, so your letter writers will have to submit their recommendations to both portals and you will have to fill out much of the same information twice.

When deciding if you should apply to one or the other, we recommend applying to both! Once you are accepted to multiple programs you can have the luxury of determining what program fits you best. Do not exclude DO programs because you feel there is a stigma against DOs. If you really do not want to be a DO, then hopefully you get accepted to an MD program. But, if that acceptance never comes, you may wish you had applied to both. Additionally, do not rule out MD programs just because you have low metrics.

Here is what Chase wrote on his secondary applications when asked "Why do you want to become an Osteopathic Physician?"

Osteopathic medicine attracts me for many reasons. The holistic approach of treating the body as interdependent components makes sense to me. I appreciate the methodology of osteopathy; considering the patient's environment, nutrition, and other factors to aid in the diagnosis and treatment of medical conditions.

Additionally, I am fascinated by manipulative medicine. The additional training that osteopaths receive compared to traditional physicians seems, to me, as a must for treating patients as effectively as possible. Physicians are supposed to do no harm; I believe that if a medical condition is treatable by manipulation, then that option should be prioritized over medication. Although not all medications are harmful to the body, it is still the physician's responsibility to provide the best care for their patients.

From my shadowing experiences of both MDs and DOs, I continuously fall more in love with osteopathic medicine. I have had allopathic physicians tell me that they wish they had considered osteopathic medical schools because of the more holistic approach and manipulative techniques. One DO physician in particular that I have shadowed made physical therapy and other non-surgical procedures a cornerstone of their practice.

To summarize, I do not think there is a single tenet that draws me to osteopathic medicine but rather the overall approach and attitude that DO physicians show toward their patients that pulls me in.

TYPES OF INTERVIEWS

If you make it to the interview stage, congratulations! This means the admissions committee likes you better than about 80% of their other applicants. The purpose of the interview is to determine if you are the best fit for their school and to weed out those who may look great on paper but would not do well interfacing with patients. It can also provide admissions committees the opportunity to ask you about potential red flags that they saw in your application.

They do not interview applicants unless they are very serious about accepting them. When it comes to interviews, they care about personality and demeanor more than anything else. This is your time to show professionalism and conversational skills. Saying the phrase "Yes sir" or "No ma'am," as well as maintaining appropriate eye contact and body language is vital for a successful interview. Since you made it to this stage, your written application is no longer a strong factor. From this point forward, it is mainly your performance during the interview that determines whether you get an acceptance letter.

There are mainly two interviewing techniques medical schools use. The most widely known method is the traditional interview. This is typically one-on-one with a professor, admissions coordinator, or physician. Some programs may also use current medical students, deans, community members, or researchers. You may have one or several interviews that can range from 15 to 60 minutes each.

Your interviewer does not always have your application beforehand, or at all! These are known as 'blind interviews.' There are many pros and cons to this interview style. For example, let's say you are a phenomenal applicant on paper but an average interviewee. If the interviewer has never seen your application, there is nothing to set you apart from someone who is not as accomplished or extraordinary as you. Though, the tables can turn if the opposite is true. You may not be the most accomplished but now you have the opportunity to impress the interviewer based on your personality and well thought out answers.

Another model of interviewing that has become very popular is Multiple Mini Interviews (MMI). You may have heard scary stories about MMI's but they are not as bad as they seem. We actually found them kind of fun. During an MMI, you shuffle through several (sometimes more than 10) interview stations. Some stations may just be very short traditional style interviews while others could be scenario-based, this is most common. Before entering the interview room, you are given a prompt for which you will form a well-constructed response. These prompts may be as easy as "Tell me a time you have embraced diversity" or could be as complex as "Imagine you work in a pharmacy. What would you do if a parent asked you to steal life-saving medication for their dying child?"

For MMI's you typically are allotted 1-2 minutes to read the prompt and form a response outside the room. You will have a piece of paper that you can gather your thoughts on and reference during the interview. Once you enter the room, you will have 5-10 minutes to explain your thoughts. The interviewer will be taking notes and usually does not have a dialogue with you. However, they may ask for you to elaborate on a point or intentionally challenge your stance, but not much more. Because this is not a back and forth conversation, you will feel awkward. This is completely normal, everyone does. For the scenario-style prompts, you will need to be very strategic regarding your answers. If you are given 8 minutes to speak, you do not want to be finished by minute 3.

There are some basic points that you should follow in MMIs. Always introduce yourself and shake hands with the interviewer upon entering the room. The interviewer may ask you if you understood the prompt, but oftentimes they will not say anything. To burn time and ensure you read the correct prompt, you should first summarize the prompt and questions being asked. Maintain eye contact and speak confidently. It is okay to glance down at your paper but try not to look at it more than the interviewer. Next, you should discuss at least two perspectives from the questions at hand. Then, if applicable, show why one point-of-view is the best, most rational option. Remain non-judgmental and empathetic throughout your response. When you are done speaking, summarize your thoughts and ask if you adequately answered the prompt's questions. This is to ensure you did not forget an aspect of the question and makes for a smoother transition if the interviewer wants you to elaborate on anything. Finally, when you are leaving, shake their hand again and thank them for their time.

MMI's can be tricky. They will throw you off your game and may ask challenging questions. But, if you can provide a well-constructed response and have a pleasant demeanor, you will be fine. Not all MMI's are the same. For example, some interviewers are instructed to try to make you change your final answer and may argue with you. This is to see how you deal with conflict. There are usually multiple "correct" answers and as long as you construct an ethical, well thought out perspective. For the most part, you should never change your answer unless you realize you said something unethical or inappropriate, which hopefully you did not. Another situation could be that the interviewer does not speak to you at all; this made us feel awkward at first and increased our stress because we were not getting any social cues. Keep calm and just know that this is all a part of the interview. Try your best to proceed with grace. Finally, you may be asked to teach simple tasks such as brushing their teeth. This is to see how well you are able to communicate. Brushing your teeth is probably a basic task for you but translate that to a routine medical procedure that you must explain to a patient in terms they understand.

While MMI's and traditional style interviews make up the majority of interview scenarios, there are other styles to be aware of. Chase had an interview with seven other applicants and two facilitators at one time. Some programs prefer panel-style; several interviewers with one interviewee. At one of our interviews, we both were surprised by a remote interviewer. This was more difficult than expected because we could not read the interviewer's body language and their responses were delayed. It was also strange to speak into a camera and then look to a screen across the room for a response.

To summarize, the interviews can be stressful. But, if you can act like a pleasant, respectable person, you probably do not have anything to worry about. With all of these different interviewing styles, there are many ways to prepare for your interview, which we will discuss in the next section.

PREPARING FOR AN INTERVIEW

Once you have received your interview invitation, congratulations, there is a medical school that wants you to attend their program! It is now up to you to affirm their beliefs that you are the person they want. Notice we said 'person' and not 'student.' If you have received an interview, they believe that you are a strong enough student to attend medical school at their institution. The interview is the first time they will have an actual conversation with you, face to face. This will show your speaking abilities, critical thinking skills, and honestly, will reveal if you are a person they would feel comfortable interfacing with patients and representing their school.

The interview should be more than just showing up and answering questions. It starts immediately after you receive an invitation. Typically, you will have to accept their offer rather quickly. This is usually through the school's admission portal website. Their website typically will have information pertaining to your application and the day you have been asked to interview. Some programs are more personal and will require you to email them back and confirm. Some programs are very blunt about when you will interview, giving you the date and time to arrive. Other programs may give you multiple dates and you get to choose when works best for you. F given the option, we believe you should try to pick the earliest date possible.

Remember, when you send an email to anyone in the admissions department, be as professional as possible. Write your emails in complete sentences, use titles like Dr., Mr., Ms., etc. Also, if you are responding to a question, use the phrase 'Yes sir, Yes ma'am.' This may make you feel uncomfortable but this shows your level of professionalism and respect.

Next, you need to determine how you are going to get there. Are you going to drive? Do you need a hotel? Make these reservations early. Many times if you need to stay in a hotel, the medical school will have a discount code made available for a specific hotel. It is also pretty common for the school's current medical students will offer interviewees a bed to stay the night before their interview at no cost. This is a great option to save some money and get the inside scoop on the program.

The night before interviews it is common for schools to host "meet and greets." This is usually a casual event with current medical students and interviewees for the next day. There may or may not be an admissions member in attendance. We never went to any of these as interviewees, mainly because we would travel to the interview the morning of (to save money), however, we help host these events at our medical school now. They are a great way to help gain insight into the medical school in a more relaxed setting. In addition, when asked during the interview why you want to attend that particular institution, you will be able to speak on the camaraderie of the current students and back-up claims that you can see yourself in their shoes next year

The dress code for medical school interviews is strict business professional. When in doubt, dress nicer than you think you should. You do not need to go out and spend a thousand dollars on an outfit but definitely take this cost into account when budgeting for the application process. For men, wear a suit. Black and navy are both safe choices. You can still stand out, a dress watch or bold tie are nice touches. If you have not purchased a suit and had it tailored, now would be the time. It was very obvious when someone was wearing a non-fitted suit. Additionally, I would recommend purchasing one nice tie. I wore the same outfit thing to every interview. I also brought a leather portfolio folder to every interview. It was nice to be able to store the goodies they gave us in there as well as lip balm and extra pens. Finally, for men, do not wear any visible piercings or tattoos if possible. Technically, schools are not supposed to discriminate on appearance, but let's be honest, they absolutely do. These details will become less of an issue as you move up in your career but you need to get there first. Do not let your appearance be the reason you are not accepted.

For women, you should also wear a suit. Black or gray are safe choices. This should be properly fitted, not too tight or too loose. You can wear pants or a skirt on the bottom with closed-toed shoes. Bring a professional purse and/or a leather portfolio folder. You can keep notepads, bandaids, snacks, pens, your keys, et cetera inside. Flats are a good choice of shoe because you will be walking all day to tour the campus. Try to break in your shoes before the interview but also bring Band-Aids because you never know when you are going to get a blister. Make-up should be kept to a minimum and nails should be of reasonable length and neutral color. You are dressing for the position that you want and you are not able to give a proper physical exam with inch-long nails. Additionally, you do not want to walk out of the interview room and have them talking about your fashion choices rather than your responses to their questions. You still have some ways to stand out. You can accessorize with reasonable jewelry and a broach. Keep piercings to a minimum and try to keep tattoos covered the best you can. As stated in the men's section, schools are not supposed to discriminate on appearance, but they definitely do. These details will become less of an issue as you move up in your career but you need to get there first. Do not let your appearance be the reason you are not accepted.

There are a few questions that are almost guaranteed to be asked during your interview. The reason they are asked so many times is because they are *that* important. Be sure to have your responses ready, just make sure you don't sound like a robot reciting what you've practiced to your bathroom mirror a dozen times.

Here is a list of questions that we have personally been asked. Think about what you would say and ask yourself if it sounds cliche or disingenuous.

- Why do you want to become a physician?
- Why become a physician and not a {nurse, physician assistant, nurse practitioner}?
- Tell me about a time where you had to make a tough decision that the rest of the group did not agree with.
- Tell me about a time you failed.
- How do you handle stress?
- Who is the most influential person in your life?
- Why are you a good fit for our medical school?
- What is your first choice of medical school?
- Why should we accept you into our medical school?
- What will you do if you are not accepted to medical school this year? Do you have an alternative career plan?
- Do you have any questions for me?

Here is a tip we have learned along the way. As stated in the question list above, admissions committees love to ask "Tell me about a time you failed." This is your opportunity to explain something from your application that may not paint you in the best light. Madeline always used this question to explain her less than desirable grades at the beginning of her college career. She explained this a bit in her personal statement but was able to elaborate more clearly and directly in the interview, explaining the steps she took to correct the problem. If you had an issue, admissions committees love to see that if you recognized it, fixed it, and learned from it.

Finally, it is okay to be stumped by a question during the interview. Just politely tell them, "That's a great question! Is it okay if I take a minute to gather my thoughts?" Do not think for literally sixty seconds, but ten seconds is perfectly acceptable. Though, if you can have much of your thoughts already organized before the interview, this will lead to a smoother day.

WHAT THE INTERVIEW DAY LOOKS LIKE

Most interview days start in the morning around 8 am or 9 am. You are typically expected to arrive between ten and thirty minutes early; the earlier the better. This allows you time to park and find the meeting location on an unfamiliar campus. It is better to wait 30 minutes for the day to start than be the last person to arrive. You are typically provided a link to print out a parking pass, or you are told a specific parking lot to park in. We recommend using Google Maps to locate the building you are going to and find the parking lot digitally, as well. This helps ensure you know exactly where you are going and do not need to worry about it the morning of.

When you arrive, you are typically greeted by an admissions member at the door and led or directed to a meeting room. There will usually be 10-20 other students present to interview as well. Oftentimes water, coffee, and light refreshments are available, but from our experience, it is best to eat breakfast on your own before you arrive. Be friendly with the other interviewees, you are all nervous and some of them could be in your class one day!

Typically, the day will consist of a guided tour of the medical campus, short lectures regarding financial aid, possibly a pop-in greeting of one of the deans, lunch with current medical students, presentations on why their school is the best, how amazing their city is, and of course the interview. Each school schedules their interview days differently so there will be some variability but almost all of our interview days consisted of the list above in some order or another.

The tour of the campus is usually around an hour and a half.

During this time, you are typically guided by an M1 or M2 (first-year or second-year medical student), though it could be an admissions member. You will be directed through the library, anatomy lab (no, you will not see any cadavers), classrooms, dining facilities, computer simulation facilities (if the program has one), academic enrichment centers (where academic advisors are typically found), and anything else pertinent to that program.

Every school will have financial aid to speak to you. They will give you advice that you will probably already know, such as take out as few loans as you can. They will also give information that you probably didn't know, such as how to apply for their school-specific scholarships and what their FAFSA (Free Application for Federal Student Aid) code is. They may also discuss alternative methods for paying for medical schools such as the military, national health service corps, or other similar programs.

The admissions committee member who is facilitating the interview day will typically have a presentation. This usually involves the curriculum, atmosphere of the school, and what their board scores typically look like. They will also talk about certain statistics that make their school look appealing such as diversity ratios, research budgets, or important alumni. Additionally, the presentation may include information about the city the school resides in and affiliated hospitals and clinics. This is usually the best time to ask specific questions regarding the academia and clinical side of the school.

The school will provide lunch for you. Only a couple of the schools we interviewed at told us in advance what would be provided or asked about dietary restrictions. So, if you are vegetarian, vegan, gluten-free, lactose intolerant, etc. do not be afraid to bring your own snacks! Many people do, it is okay! We were provided anything from pizza, to wraps, to chipotle. One of the schools we interviewed at allotted us $10 to the school's cafeteria!

These are very long days and you will be tired by the end. Just be sure to stay professional and polite all day but definitely take advantage of the freebie they provide! Madeline may or may not have eaten seven packets of fruit snacks between interviews.

THANK YOU LETTERS

Once you complete your interview day and leave to travel home, the process for you is not over. There is a critical step many people fail to complete. You must send thank you cards to your interviewers! This is critical in showing your professionalism as well as your desire to attend their program. The letter does not have to be extremely formal but it should be written on a physical card and mailed. Some people may feel like an email is sufficient, but go the extra step and send a physical note. This makes it more personal, and honestly, who doesn't like to receive handwritten letters in the mail? Some schools will provide you with the names of your interviewers, especially if you only have two or three. If not, it is okay to send the note to the admissions department. Here are the thank you letters Chase used, but feel free to make yours your own:

Dear (School) Admissions Staff,
I just wanted to reach out to you and express my gratitude for taking the time to show me your incredible campus. I felt at home and can honestly see myself there. I enjoyed meeting and interacting not only with the admissions committee but with the students as well. I truly felt the sense of community between the students and the faculty. I hope I am able to come and visit you again in (City)!
Sincerely,
First Last

Dear Dr. (Last name),
I just wanted to reach out to you and express my gratitude for taking the time to meet with me. The sense of community between the students and the faculty was evident throughout my visit and I felt right at home. I hope I am able to meet with you again.

Sincerely,
First Last

Dear (Student's name),
I just wanted to reach out to you and express my gratitude for taking the time to meet with me. I really appreciate you answering all my questions, specifically about the new curriculum and how classes work. Good luck with your board studying!
Sincerely,
First Last

HOW TO CHOOSE BETWEEN MEDICAL SCHOOLS

Congratulations, you have been accepted to a medical school! Hopefully, you have been accepted to multiple programs and now have the fortunate burden of determining which school is the best fit for you. We have discussed several differences between schools throughout the book so far, but this section is advice on how to narrow down your options to one program.

The best place to begin is before you were even selected. After every interview you attend, you should reflect on your experience and write down your thoughts. This will help you several months down the line when you have attended several different interviews and they all blend together. This does not need to be in immaculate detail but should cover important factors *for you*. For us, this included what the expectations are for in-class attendance, how the anatomy lab is run, how long your dedicated board exam study period is, third-year rotation schedule and options, clinical-setting preparation, and just general atmosphere. You will learn many things during your interview about the school that was not explicitly stated on the website, so write them down! You may learn that one program has mandatory classes four hours a day five days a week, and another program only has 4 hours of mandatory events every other week. Trust us when we say, the fewer mandatory events you have to go to the better.

The next factor that should be considered is the location. Some programs are located in the middle of nowhere, others may be in the middle of a large city. Different locations have different benefits, it all depends on your personal preference as well as the potential for exposure to diverse patient populations.

The size of your class will also have some impact on your education. There are programs with almost 300 students per class and others that have less than 20. I'm sure you can see the education you would receive from those schools would be quite different. This is completely up to you, there are benefits to both cohort sizes as well as drawbacks.

One factor that we feel should only be slightly considered is cost. Medical school is expensive. Some programs are *ridiculously* expensive, but for the most part, do not let the cost of a program prevent you from attending your dream school.

For the most part, choosing your future home for the next four years is a massive decision. If we were in the position to choose a medical school over again, knowing what we know now, we would choose a large MD program in an urban area that gives students the most freedom with the least amount of mandatory work.

THE GAME OF CHANCE

Unfortunately, even if you did everything perfectly, there is still the element of chance in determining your fate. Human nature and emotion are involved and the person reading your primary application could have had a horrible fight with their significant other or even have a bias toward people who share your first name! They could have read the most incredible application they have ever seen right before your moderately-awesome application. Love it or hate it, the application process has flaws. Many programs have implemented protocols and computer systems to help minimize these types of unfair decisions. But, to reduce the risk of bad luck, you should send your application to 12-20 programs.

The best way to improve your chances is to have a perfect application. Sounds impossible? Well, that's because it is. Just do your best and do not give the admissions committee any extra ammunition to shoot down your application. Write a flawless personal statement, dress professionally, and do not have any violations. You want to look as appealing and low-risk as possible.

SECTION THREE:

You Didn't Get Accepted or You're Taking a Gap Year

OVERVIEW OF SECTION THREE

This section is all about gap years. Some people may intentionally postpone their application to allow them to have a year 'off.' Others are unfortunately forced into one, either by not gaining an acceptance or other reasons. The good news is, gap years are beneficial for many reasons. Though, this is a double edged-sword. You have the luxury of taking a year to buff up your CV and become a much more competitive applicant, but you are postponing a year of your education. One year may not seem that long, but when you think about how long your medical education takes, you may want to start earlier rather than later.

Regardless of how you may have ended up in a gap year, the question is now, "What do I do?"

RESEARCH

Almost every person that takes a gap year will participate in some form of research. This is one of those things that can only benefit you. It is a *permanent* addition to your CV, and will make you more competitive not only for applying to medical school, but for residency and fellowships as well.

Research is also one of the easiest activities to get involved with. If you participated in research in undergrad, you can try to rejoin a project or use those connections to help find another project. It is also fairly common to find research opportunities on LinkedIn. Spend some time researching faculty members at nearby universities, as well. Try to find projects that interest you, particularly those that involve a field of medicine you may be interested in. You can also ask physicians whom you are familiar with if they have any projects they are working on or know of any that you may be able to join.

A word to the wise, medical schools, residencies, and fellowships tend to value quantity rather than quality. Though this is not always true, such as if you can get published in The New England Journal of Medicine or another well-known journal that carries a large amount of weight. But realistically, the odds of obtaining something that prestigious is quite small. Try to focus on projects that are likely to provide several publications.

GET A JOB

Another common path to take during a gap year is getting a job. We would strongly encourage you, if you choose this path, to get a job working for a physician or hospital. This will give you experience in the healthcare field and will look much more appealing on your CV than working in a non-medical environment.

We have many peers who worked as scribes, nurses assistants, EMTs, or patient care advocates. These look great on your medical school application! It shows your dedication to medicine and that you have experienced the medical field from the inside. Not to mention gaining invaluable clinical knowledge that will become second nature to you by the time you start medical school.

Our favorite, but perhaps most difficult to attain, job would be working for a physician who owns their own practice. Many of these independently owned practices are super willing to hire pre-med students, particularly those taking gap years. This is our favorite option if you do decide to get a job. Not only will you be working closely with a physician, but you are very likely to get a great letter of recommendation as well. Again, it will provide you with invaluable clinical experience that will give you an edge in medical school. Finally, that physician will most likely know some members of the selections committees for nearby medical schools. This personal connection could be that extra boost you need when it comes to reapplying.

ENJOY YOUR TIME, BUT NOT TOO MUCH

You should enjoy your time away from school! Spend time with friends and family, travel to places you've always wanted to go, and just grow as a person. Once you go back to school you are much more limited in your free time and your schedule quickly fills up. Now, this does not mean that you should only relax and travel. You should continue to build your CV. Admissions committees will most definitely ask you how your spent your gap year, and leisurely traveling the entire time is unfortunately not the answer they want to hear.

Furthermore, it is imperative that you do not get in trouble with the law. Gap years can be a great asset if managed properly. Having a run-in with the legal system can be one of the fastest ways to end your medical career. We don't want to sound like your mother, but just don't put yourself in situations where you can get into trouble and do not associate with bad influences. This seems simple enough but sadly many future healthcare hopefuls fall into this category. Think about it this way, what do you want medical school admissions committees to find when they google your name? A news article of you volunteering at a free clinic or an article on your recent arrest?

YOU (MOST LIKELY) DON'T HAVE TO RETAKE THE MCAT

More often than not, the first thing people do when they do not get accepted into medical school is blame their MCAT scores. Yes, it is true that your MCAT score was probably lower than you were hoping for (most people's were). However, retaking your MCAT will probably not help your application as much as you think. It is not uncommon to get the same, or even a lower score. You will probably stress yourself out studying for the exam and, above all, you will only be focusing on one aspect of your application. Use this time to build your CV! It is worth more to gain experience in the field; volunteer, shadow, get a job, and assist in research rather than hope to improve one single factor of your application.

We know many people who were not accepted, immediately started to study for the MCAT, and received calls offering acceptances into programs late in the cycle (May, June, and July). In addition, every time you take the MCAT, the schools you apply to see each of your scores. For example, if you take the MCAT three times, medical schools will see all three of your scores. Some schools may even average your scores. So, unless you score an extraordinarily high score, it will not matter that much anyway.

We would only recommend retaking your MCAT if you scored less than a 495. Even then, we still feel like you have a decent chance of getting accepted if you can build the rest of your application over your gap year. When in doubt, your MCAT is *not* worth retaking!

GO BACK TO SCHOOL

Due to the increasingly competitive nature of medical school admissions, many students are matriculating into medical school having already completed some level of postgraduate education. This could be as simple as completing a few courses over a semester pertaining to science or even business. More commonly, applicants may consider master's programs. One such program is a master's of anatomy and physiology.

These programs are typically offered at universities that also have medical schools. Thus, you will take the same professors, or even the same exact courses, as the medical students. This will greatly prepare you for the anatomy and physiology of medical school as well as give you a massive leg up when applying to that program. These degrees are valued highly when applying and provide incredible networking opportunities.

Another option, which has been written about in detail earlier in this book, is pipeline master's programs. To illustrate what these programs look like, we will give an example. Our good friend, like many, was unfortunately not accepted into a medical school on his first attempt. So he decided to look into medical school pipeline programs. The program he was accepted into was not as competitive as medical school, but at a renowned institution that many us of can only dream of attending. During his one year program, he took many of the same courses that the first-year medical students take, worked in a couple of research labs, had his name added to several publications, and was guaranteed an interview at that school's corresponding medical school. He happily held a seat in their medical school program just one year later.

These programs are offered at the majority of medical schools.

Unfortunately, many students are unaware of them because they are not highly publicized. Roughly 10% of our medical school class came from the pipeline program. If you have decided that you want to return to education to better your chances for matriculating, we would recommend finding a program that has ties to a medical school with a guaranteed interview following the completion of their program.

STILL WANT MORE INFORMATION?

First of all, thank you for reading this book! We spent hundreds of hours brainstorming and writing to elaborate on as many topics as we could think of. Though, if you are anything like us, you want all the information you can get!

We encourage you to check out our YouTube channel, *Maddie x Chase*. We create videos that are related to the pre-medical experience, applying to medical school, and what medical school is actually like. As we're sure you know by now, we try our best to keep things genuine and honest. We are sure that this resource will only continue to grow with our education.

If you want to connect with us, YouTube is the best place to do so! Comment or message us through our page and we will try our best to respond. If we do not already have a video on the topic you are curious about, we will make one!

Again, thank you for taking the time to read our book. It means a lot to us and we are honored to play a part in your medical journey. Best of luck to you, Future Doctor.

www.ingramcontent.com/pod-product-compliance
Lightning Source LLC
Chambersburg PA
CBHW031448210526
45464CB00005B/2368